PREDIABETES DIET PLAN

A Busy Professional's Step-by-Step Guide
to Managing Prediabetes Through Diet

Brandon Gilta

mindplusfood

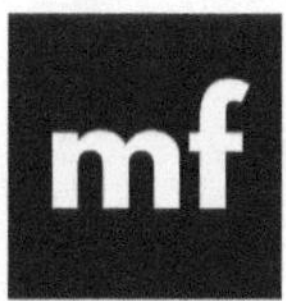

DISCLAIMER

By reading this disclaimer, you are accepting the terms of the disclaimer in full. If you disagree with this disclaimer, please do not read the guide.

All of the content within this guide is provided for informational and educational purposes only, and should not be accepted as independent medical or other professional advice. The author is not a doctor, physician, nurse, mental health provider, or registered nutritionist/dietician. Therefore, using and reading this guide does not establish any form of a physician-patient relationship.

Always consult with a physician or another qualified health provider with any issues or questions you might have regarding any sort of medical condition. Do not ever disregard any qualified professional medical advice or delay seeking that advice because of anything you have read in this guide. The information in this guide is not intended to be any sort of medical advice and should not be used in lieu of any medical advice by a licensed and qualified medical professional.

The information in this guide has been compiled from a variety of known sources. However, the author cannot attest to or guarantee the accuracy of each source and thus should not be held liable for any errors or omissions.

You acknowledge that the publisher of this guide will not be held liable for any loss or damage of any kind incurred as a result of this guide or the reliance on any information provided within this guide. You acknowledge and agree that you assume all risk and responsibility for any action you undertake in response to the information in this guide.

Using this guide does not guarantee any particular result (e.g., weight loss or a cure). By reading this guide, you acknowledge that there are no guarantees to any specific outcome or results you can expect.

All product names, diet plans, or names used in this guide are for identification purposes only and are the property of their respective owners. The use of these names does not imply endorsement. All other trademarks cited herein are the property of their respective owners.

Where applicable, this guide is not intended to be a substitute for the original work of this diet plan and is, at most, a supplement to the original work for this diet plan and never a direct substitute. This guide is a personal expression of the facts of that diet plan.

Where applicable, persons shown in the cover images are stock photography models and the publisher has obtained the rights to use the images through license agreements with third-party stock image companies.

CONTENTS

INTRODUCTION

As we go about our daily lives, it's easy to overlook the impact that our food choices have on our health. Yet now more than ever, it's become increasingly clear that what we eat plays a crucial role in determining our overall wellness. For those diagnosed with prediabetes—a condition where blood sugar levels are higher than normal, but not yet high enough to be classified as type 2 diabetes—paying attention to the food we eat is especially important. Making healthy dietary choices can be daunting, but when it comes to preventing the onset of type 2 diabetes, a nutritious diet is one of the best ways to improve your overall health.

Prediabetes is a widespread condition that affects millions of Americans today. According to the Centers for Disease Control and Prevention (CDC), more than 84 million people in the United States currently have prediabetes—and a staggering 90% of them are unaware that they have it. This lack of awareness is a significant problem, as untreated prediabetes can eventually lead to type 2 diabetes, a potentially life-threatening condition. The good news is that prediabetes can often be reversed through a combination of lifestyle changes, including dietary adjustments.

So what does a prediabetes diet entail? Simply put, it involves making healthier food choices that help to stabilize blood sugar levels and reduce the risk of type 2 diabetes. The first step is to cut back on processed foods, refined sugars, and carbohydrates, which can cause blood sugar spikes and contribute to insulin resistance. Instead, focus on incorporating more whole grains, fresh fruits and vegetables, lean proteins, and healthy fats into your diet. These foods are lower in calories and higher in fiber, vitamins, and nutrients, making them ideal choices for those looking to improve their overall health.

Research has shown that a diet rich in whole foods can significantly reduce the risk of developing type 2 diabetes. A study published in the New England Journal of Medicine found that people with prediabetes who followed a specially designed diet and exercise program were able to reduce their risk of progressing to type 2 diabetes by over 50% compared to those who made no changes to their lifestyle. Another study published in the journal Diabetes Care found that a diet rich in fruits, vegetables, whole grains, and low-fat dairy products was associated with a lower risk of developing type 2 diabetes.

Of course, making dietary changes can be challenging, especially in a world where junk food and processed snacks are ubiquitous. But the benefits of a healthy diet are undeniable—not only can it help to prevent type 2 diabetes, but it can also reduce the risk of other health problems like heart disease, stroke, and certain types of cancer. And with the right tools and support, anyone can make positive changes to their eating habits.

In this guide, we'll explore the ins and outs of a prediabetes diet, from the foods to eat (and avoid) to practical strategies for making healthy eating a part of your daily routine. We'll also provide a 5-step guide on how to get started with a prediabetes diet and some meal recipes that you can try out. Read on to learn more about the power of nutrition and how you can use it to manage your health.

WHAT IS PREDIABETES?

Prediabetes is a stage in which you have sugar levels that are high enough to alarm your doctor, but not high enough to be considered diabetes. You are at a crossroads.

Interestingly, 5 to 10% of the overall population develops prediabetes. It does not seem so bad. However, with the types of food that are being offered and sold in shops and restaurants today, you can bet that the numbers can still escalate. When you do end up being part of the statistics, things are a little tougher. 70% of people with prediabetes develop full-blown diabetes. This is a scary outlook. However, you can look at the bright side: you can still attempt to be part of the 30% that do turn their blood sugar levels around.

While there is hope, you have to take things seriously. A prediabetes diagnosis can be tough. There are underlying issues that you have to tackle, such as a genetic predisposition or insulin resistance.

Prediabetes usually does not have symptoms. So, if you have moved on to the increased thirst, constant hunger, blurred vision, and fatigue territory, you may already have diabetes. Your mission, with the help of this guide, is to avoid getting to that level.

Factors that Make You Susceptible to Prediabetes and Diabetes
It is important to understand the factors that make you more susceptible to prediabetes and diabetes. These include genetics, age, sex, ethnicity, family history of diabetes, lifestyle choices such as diet and physical activity levels, weight gain, or obesity.

1. Poor diet: Regular consumption of unhealthy foods, high in sugar and saturated fats, can increase the risk of developing prediabetes and diabetes. This is because consuming too much sugar and unhealthy fats can cause blood glucose levels to rise significantly, putting a strain on the pancreas and liver. These organs are responsible for regulating insulin production and maintaining proper glucose levels in the body. Therefore, it is essential to limit the intake of such foods and focus on a healthier and balanced diet to prevent the onset of prediabetes and diabetes. Making smarter food choices and adopting a healthy and active lifestyle can help individuals avoid these health risks and ensure optimal well-being.

2. Lack of physical activity: Living a sedentary lifestyle with little to no physical activity can have adverse effects on one's health. Not only does it decrease muscle mass, but it also reduces insulin sensitivity, leading to an increased risk of metabolic diseases such as prediabetes and diabetes. A sedentary lifestyle is a lifestyle that is counterproductive to physical health. Consistent exercise can increase muscle mass and improve insulin sensitivity, making it an effective way to prevent metabolic diseases. By incorporating physical activity into daily life, individuals can improve their overall health and decrease their vulnerability to metabolic diseases. The benefits of exercise are numerous, and it is never too late to start engaging in physical activity.

3. Genetics: Type 2 diabetes is a complex and multifactorial disease that is influenced by both genetic and environmental factors. If there is a family history of type 2 diabetes, then the risk of developing the disease increases significantly. This means that certain genes that predispose an individual to type 2 diabetes

may have been passed down from generation to generation. While genetics do play a role in the development of the disease, it is important to note that lifestyle factors such as diet and exercise also contribute to the onset of diabetes. Individuals with a family history of type 2 diabetes need to be aware of their increased risk and take proactive measures to manage their health. Maintaining a healthy lifestyle and seeking medical advice can help to prevent or delay the onset of this disease.

4. Age: As the years go by, the human body undergoes a range of changes that can increase the risk for prediabetes and type 2 diabetes. It's not just about genetics or lifestyle choices. As we age, our insulin sensitivity drops, making our bodies less responsive to this vital hormone. Additionally, our metabolism slows down, contributing to changes in blood sugar levels. Finally, hormonal imbalances associated with aging can make it more difficult for the body to regulate glucose in the blood. By staying informed about the risks associated with aging and taking proactive steps, we can help reduce the risk of developing diabetes in our later years.

5. Weight: Maintaining a healthy weight is crucial in preventing prediabetes and type 2 diabetes. Being overweight or obese can have a serious impact on insulin sensitivity, leading to elevated blood glucose levels. This harmful cycle can increase the likelihood of developing diabetes over time. To break this cycle, it's important to prioritize a healthy diet and exercise routine. By making small, sustainable changes to your lifestyle, you can significantly reduce your risk of developing diabetes and improve your overall health. Take control of your weight and take control of your health.

6. Stress: It's no secret that stress takes a toll on our bodies, both mentally and physically. But did you know that prolonged periods of stress can disrupt the delicate balance of hormones in our bodies? This disruption can cause an increase in glucose levels, which, over time, may increase the risk of developing diabetes. It's

important to take measures to manage stress levels to maintain overall health and well-being. Whether it's through physical activity, relaxation techniques, or seeking professional support, taking steps to combat stress can have a profound impact on our bodies and our lives.

7. Gender: When it comes to gestational diabetes, women are unfortunately at a higher risk than men. This condition can have serious consequences if not managed properly, and it often serves as a warning sign for the future development of type 2 diabetes. Despite common misconceptions, women tend to gain weight more easily than men, which only adds to their chances of experiencing prediabetes and diabetes. It's important for women who are pregnant or planning to become pregnant to be proactive about their health to mitigate these risks. By staying informed and taking steps to manage their weight and blood sugar levels, women can reduce the likelihood of developing gestational diabetes and safeguard their long-term health.

8. Ethnicity: Certain ethnicities are at a higher risk for developing prediabetes and type 2 diabetes compared with others. This increased susceptibility can stem from a combination of genetic and cultural factors that impact diet, exercise habits, and healthcare accessibility. While notable advancements have been made in diabetes prevention and treatment, it is important to recognize and address these disparities so that all individuals have equal access to preventative care and resources. By prioritizing awareness and working to address these gaps, we can ensure that everyone has the opportunity to live a healthy and vibrant life regardless of their background.

9. Smoking: Smoking has been found to have a significant impact on one's health, specifically when it comes to type 2 diabetes. Studies have shown that smokers are more likely than nonsmokers to develop this chronic condition. The reason for this lies in the way cigarette smoke affects the body. The smoke can weaken peripheral nerves responsible for controlling

blood glucose levels, leading to metabolic dysfunction and pre-diabetic states. Moreover, it can also have adverse effects on the cardiovascular system, further exacerbating the risk of developing type 2 diabetes. To mitigate this risk, it is crucial for smokers to quit and for nonsmokers to avoid exposure to cigarette smoke wherever possible. By doing so, we can all work to ensure that our bodies are healthy and functioning at their best.

10. Drugs/Medications: Recent studies have revealed that several commonly prescribed drugs can have unwanted side effects on your body's insulin levels, ultimately leading to pre-diabetes. Certain medications used to treat high cholesterol, hypertension, depression, and schizophrenia have been linked to decreased insulin sensitivity, meaning that your body may not be able to use insulin effectively. Moreover, some HIV medications have been shown to cause significant weight gain, ultimately increasing the risk of developing diabetes if not properly monitored. It's essential to educate yourself on the potential risks associated with any medication you take and work closely with a healthcare professional to mitigate any harmful effects. Remember, prevention is always better than cure!

11. Alcohol Consumption: Studies have revealed that heavy drinking regularly is not only bad for the liver, but also increases the possibility of developing pre-diabetes and diabetes. Alcohol is a sneaky culprit, affecting our body's metabolism in ways that are often overlooked. It interferes with the body's ability to regulate insulin and blood sugar levels, leading to cellular stress and inflammation. While moderate alcohol consumption may not pose a significant risk, it's important to be mindful of our drinking habits and limit excessive alcohol consumption to reduce the risk of developing diabetes.

12. Sleep Deprivation: Sleep deprivation can have severe consequences on our body, including an increased risk of developing prediabetes and diabetes. Studies have shown that a lack of restorative sleep can cause fluctuations in glucose levels

and insulin resistance, leading to these conditions. Chronic sleep deprivation can disrupt the hormones responsible for regulating blood sugar levels, leading to adverse effects on insulin sensitivity. It is up to individuals to prioritize sleep and create a sustainable sleep routine that allows for a sufficient amount of restorative sleep to avoid such health-related consequences. By getting adequate sleep, it is possible to take a proactive approach to managing one's health and preventing the onset of diabetes.

Having an understanding of these risk factors is essential to create an effective plan for managing your health and reducing the risk of developing type 2 diabetes.

Complications of Prediabetes

While it is important to be aware of the risk factors associated with type 2 diabetes, it is also essential to understand the potential complications that can arise from prediabetes. Here are some of the potential complications:

● High Blood Pressure: If you have prediabetes, it is important to be aware of the potential complications that may arise, one of which is high blood pressure. Prediabetes means that your blood sugar levels are higher than normal, but not yet high enough to be classified as diabetes. However, even at this pre-diabetic stage, your body can already experience negative effects. When your blood sugar levels are elevated, your body retains salt and water, leading to an increase in blood pressure.

● Heart Disease: If you have prediabetes and have difficulty managing your blood sugar levels, you may be at risk for developing heart disease. High blood sugar levels cause damage to the small blood vessels in your heart, leading to an increased risk of cardiovascular problems.

● Neuropathy: If you have prediabetes and don't manage it well, you greatly increase your risk of developing neuropathy, a serious condition that affects the nerves throughout your body. This is because high blood sugar levels, which are often present in unmanaged prediabetes, can gradually cause damage to these nerves, leading to pain, numbness, and weakness in different areas of your body. Over time, neuropathy can also impact your digestive system, heart, and sexual function, making it all the more important to take your prediabetes seriously and seek medical help right away.

• Kidney Disease: Prediabetes can still cause significant damage to your kidneys, as high blood sugar can damage the tiny filters in your kidneys that help remove waste products from your bloodstream. This damage can lead to a buildup of waste products in your bloodstream, which can have serious health consequences. To prevent kidney disease, it's important to manage your blood sugar levels through a healthy diet, regular exercise, and medication if necessary. You should also have regular check-ups with your doctor to monitor your kidney function and catch any problems early.

• Blindness: If you have prediabetes and leave it uncontrolled, serious complications may arise, especially in your eyes. Diabetes can alter the structure of your eyes' capillaries, leading to a medical condition called diabetic retinopathy. This condition can put you at risk of vision problems and even blindness. If you're experiencing blurry vision, sudden vision loss, or seeing spots in your visual field, talk to your healthcare provider right away. You may be prescribed medication, undergo laser therapy, or need surgery to prevent further damage to your vision. Remember that early detection is crucial, and managing your prediabetes effectively can reduce your risk of developing diabetic retinopathy and other complications.

• Stroke: Having prediabetes can put you at risk for many health complications. Among these complications is a higher risk for stroke because high blood sugar can damage your arteries. When your arteries become damaged, they become less elastic and less flexible, making it difficult for blood to flow through them. This puts a strain on your heart, causing it to work harder to pump blood throughout your body. When your arteries become clogged with plaque or clots, the blood flow to your brain can become interrupted, leading to a stroke. It's important to keep your blood sugar levels in check and maintain a healthy lifestyle to prevent the risk of stroke and other complications associated with prediabetes.

• Amputation: If you have prediabetes, you are at an increased risk of developing poor circulation in your feet. This is because high blood sugar levels can damage your blood vessels and nerves, leading to reduced blood flow to your feet. When your feet do not receive enough blood, they become more prone to developing ulcers and infections. If an infection does not respond well to treatment, amputation may be necessary. About 60% of non-traumatic lower limb amputations in the United States are due to prediabetes or diabetes. It is essential to maintain proper foot care and monitor your blood sugar levels to prevent such complications. This includes inspecting your feet daily, wearing comfortable and supportive shoes, exercising regularly, and seeing a healthcare provider for any foot problems. Remember, taking care of your feet is an essential part of managing prediabetes and preventing complications.

• Pregnancy Complications: If you have prediabetes and become pregnant, you may face various complications during pregnancy. One of the most common complications is gestational diabetes, which can put you and your baby at risk of developing type 2 diabetes later in life. Gestational diabetes can also lead to problems during delivery, such as preterm labor, preeclampsia, and cesarean section. Additionally, having prediabetes while pregnant can increase the risk of your baby developing fetal macrosomia or a larger-than-average baby. This can lead to difficulties during delivery and increase the risk of birth injuries. To prevent these complications, it is important to manage your prediabetes with a healthy diet, regular exercise, and close monitoring by your healthcare provider throughout your pregnancy.

● Skin Complications: Another complication of prediabetes is the increased risk of developing bacterial or yeast infections that can be difficult to treat. This occurs due to the high levels of glucose in the blood, which can provide a favorable environment for bacterial and fungal growth. These infections can affect various parts of the body, including the skin on the feet, hands, and genitals. It is essential to maintain good hygiene practices and keep the affected areas clean and dry. If you notice any signs of infections, such as redness, itching, or discharge, consult a healthcare provider immediately. Early detection and proper treatment can help prevent further complications.

Prediabetes and diabetes can have severe consequences on our health, from an increased risk of cardiovascular disease to potential complications during pregnancy. Therefore, it's important to be aware of the risk factors associated with type 2 diabetes and take proactive steps toward managing your health.

Preventions and Lifestyle Changes

Now that we know the primary risk factors for prediabetes, it is important to understand how we can reduce the chances of developing this chronic condition. Making simple lifestyle changes and following a healthy diet are two of the most effective ways to do so. Here are some tips that may help:

1. Balanced diet: To prevent the development of prediabetes or diabetes, you should focus on maintaining a balanced diet. This means making choices that are rich in whole grains, vegetables, and fruits, as these foods are rich in fiber, vitamins, and minerals. Additionally, you should aim to consume lean proteins, such as fish, chicken, and lentils, while limiting your intake of processed foods and sugary drinks. By avoiding foods that are high in saturated and trans fats, you can help reduce your risk of developing chronic conditions like heart disease and stroke, which are closely associated with the development of diabetes.

2. Exercise: It is important to maintain an active lifestyle to

prevent prediabetes and diabetes. Exercise should be a priority, with a minimum of 150 minutes of moderate activity or 75 minutes of vigorous activity per week. Engaging in physical activities such as walking, running, swimming, or cycling, as well as resistance training, can be beneficial. A sedentary lifestyle can increase the risk of developing prediabetes or diabetes, as well as other health problems. Regular exercise can help control blood glucose levels, improve insulin sensitivity, reduce body fat, and prevent complications associated with prediabetes and diabetes. It is important to find physical activities that you enjoy so that you can maintain a consistent exercise routine. So, incorporate exercise into your daily routine and take small steps towards a more active lifestyle to lead a healthier life.

3. Stress management: If you want to prevent developing prediabetes or diabetes, managing your stress levels is crucial. High-stress levels can lead to increased blood sugar levels, so it's important to find ways to relax and lower your stress levels. You might consider practicing mindfulness or relaxation techniques like meditation, yoga, or deep breathing exercises to help calm your mind and reduce stress. Listening to music is also a great way to unwind and alleviate stress. Research has shown that these activities can lower blood pressure, reduce cortisol levels and improve insulin sensitivity, which can help you prevent developing prediabetes or diabetes. So make sure you set aside time each day to engage in stress-reducing activities and stay on top of your health.

4. Quit smoking: Taking control of your lifestyle can significantly reduce the risk of developing prediabetes and diabetes. Quitting smoking is one key lifestyle change you can make to help protect yourself against developing these conditions. Smoking not only increases your risk for numerous health problems, but it also reduces your body's ability to process sugar properly, which in turn can increase your risk of developing prediabetes and type 2 diabetes. Quitting smoking also has immediate effects on your health, such as better lung function and improved circulation.

Speak with a doctor about strategies to quit smoking if needed. By taking this proactive step towards healthier living, you can help reduce your risk for these potentially life-threatening diseases.

5. Maintain a healthy weight: To prevent the development of prediabetes and diabetes, maintaining a healthy weight should be at the top of your priorities. Carrying excess body fat can cause your body to struggle with controlling your blood sugar levels effectively, increasing your chances of developing these conditions. Fortunately, with some simple lifestyle changes, you can take control of your weight and significantly reduce your risk of prediabetes and diabetes. Speak with a qualified dietician or nutritionist who can design a personalized meal plan that will provide you with the optimal balance of nutrients to reach your target weight safely and effectively. By implementing a healthy diet, alongside regular exercise, you can achieve a healthy weight and help prevent prediabetes or diabetes, allowing you to live a long and healthy life.

6. Get enough sleep: Lack of sleep can disrupt your body's insulin production and increase your risk of obesity, one of the leading causes of type 2 diabetes. Aim to get at least 8 hours of quality sleep each night by establishing a regular sleep schedule and avoiding caffeine and electronics before bedtime. You can also improve your sleep quality by creating a comfortable sleep environment, such as maintaining a cool temperature and using comfortable pillows and bedding. It's important to prioritize sleep in your lifestyle to maintain good health and reduce your risk of developing prediabetes or diabetes, so make sure to make changes as necessary to ensure a good night's rest. Limit alcohol intake: Limiting alcohol consumption is also important since excessive drinking can increase the risk of these conditions as well as other health problems. Speak with a doctor about how much alcohol is considered safe for you to consume to reduce your risk.

By following these tips and making lifestyle changes, it is possible to reduce the risk of developing prediabetes and diabetes. It is important to note that while making healthy choices can help prevent these conditions, regular screening is still recommended for early detection in case preventive measures fail. Speak with a doctor about your risk factors to determine an appropriate screening schedule.

A 5-STEP GUIDE BEFORE GETTING STARTED WITH PREDIABETES DIET

Now that we've discussed the risk factors and lifestyle changes that can help reduce the chances of developing prediabetes, it is important to understand how to create an effective plan for managing your health.

A good place to start is by following a prediabetes diet. This type of diet focuses on eating healthy foods, limiting processed foods and sugary drinks, and getting adequate physical activity to maintain blood sugar levels within a safe range. In this chapter, we will look at five steps you should take before beginning a prediabetes diet so that you can make sure you are setting yourself up for success from the very start.

These steps include speaking with your doctor about any dietary restrictions; calculating your daily calorie needs; understanding which food groups are beneficial; creating meal plans and grocery lists; and tracking progress along the way. By taking these measures, you will be able to ensure that you have everything in place necessary for achieving optimal results with your new eating habits.

Step 1: Speak with your Doctor
When it comes to prediabetes, lifestyle changes can play a crucial role in managing and even reversing the condition. However, before you start making any major changes to your diet, you must speak with your doctor first. Your doctor will be able to provide personalized recommendations based on your specific needs and health status. This will help ensure that you're making safe and effective choices when it comes to your food intake.

It's important to note that prediabetes can be quite complex and requires a holistic approach to management. Your doctor may recommend a variety of lifestyle changes in addition to dietary modifications, such as increasing physical activity or losing weight. By working with your doctor, you'll be able to receive guidance and support as you make these changes, which can be especially helpful if you're feeling overwhelmed or uncertain about how to get started.

Step 2: Calculate Daily Calorie Needs
Before diving into a prediabetes diet plan, it's crucial to calculate your daily calorie needs. This step is essential to ensure that you're consuming the right amount of calories based on your activity level and overall health goals. By doing so, you'll be able to develop a meal plan and grocery list tailored to your specific needs.

Calculating your daily calorie needs isn't a one-size-fits-all approach. Factors such as age, gender, weight, height, and physical activity level play a significant role in determining your daily calorie needs. For example, a moderately active 40-year-old woman who weighs 150 pounds may need more calories than a sedentary 70-year-old woman who weighs the same.

Various online calculators and apps make it easy to determine your daily calorie needs. These tools use algorithms that factor in your biological characteristics and level of activity to calculate the number of calories you need to maintain, gain, or lose weight. Once you have this information, you can plan your meals accordingly to ensure that you're consuming the appropriate amount of calories for your body.

It's important to note that consuming too few calories is just as harmful as consuming too many. Undereating can lead to malnutrition, weakness, and a compromised immune system. Therefore, it's essential to find your daily calorie needs and create a healthy meal plan. Knowing how many calories you need each day will guide you toward achieving optimal health and will help you manage prediabetes effectively.

Step 3: Understand Beneficial Foods

Before embarking on a prediabetes diet, it is crucial to understand the foods that can provide the maximum benefit to your health. The first step is to gather information from credible sources like online resources or talk to a nutritionist or your doctor to get professional advice on food choices tailored to your specific needs. It is vital to include the right kind of foods that would meet your health objectives without becoming a hindrance.

You should aim to incorporate nutrient-dense foods like whole grains, lean proteins, fruits, and vegetables into your diet. These foods are rich in essential vitamins and minerals that provide optimal nutrition, unlike processed foods that contain added sugars, saturated fats, and sodium. Nutrient-dense foods help regulate blood sugar levels, reduce inflammation, and improve overall health. Incorporating these foods into your diet, coupled with moderate exercise or physical activity, is an excellent way to manage prediabetes and prevent its progression to full-blown diabetes.

Furthermore, you should avoid foods that contain high amounts of sugar, refined carbohydrates, and unhealthy fats. Such foods spike blood sugar levels and insulin response, which can lead to insulin resistance, a hallmark of prediabetes. Therefore, choosing a balanced, nutrient-rich diet is essential to manage prediabetes effectively. By starting with this step, you can create a sustainable lifestyle that would improve your health outcomes in the long run.

Step 4: Create Meal Plans & Grocery Lists

It's important to spend some time planning out your meals and creating a grocery list. This may seem like a daunting task at first, but it's a crucial step toward achieving your health goals. By taking the time to create a meal plan ahead of time, you're setting yourself up for success and making it much easier to stick to healthier options.

When creating your meal plan, start by thinking about what types of foods will be most beneficial for your specific health needs. For those with prediabetes, it's important to focus on foods that will help stabilize blood sugar levels and minimize insulin resistance. This might include plenty of fresh vegetables, lean proteins, and healthy fats.

Once you have a general idea of what kinds of foods you'll be eating, it's time to start putting together specific meal ideas. Consider things like portion sizes, cooking methods, and flavor profiles to keep things interesting and varied. And don't forget to include healthy snack options to keep you satisfied between meals.

Finally, put together a detailed grocery list based on your meal plan. This will help ensure that you have all the ingredients on hand when it's time to cook, reducing the temptation to order takeout or rely on less healthy options.

Step 5: Track Progress

Tracking progress is essential because it allows you to identify what is working and what is not. For example, if you notice that your blood sugar levels are still high despite your efforts to eat healthier and exercise regularly, you may need to adjust your diet and exercise routine accordingly. By tracking progress, you can also celebrate your successes, no matter how small they may be. This can be a great motivator to keep going when the going gets tough.

Tracking progress doesn't have to be complicated or time-consuming. You can use a simple notebook or smartphone app to keep track of your food intake, physical activity, weight, and blood sugar levels. You can also consider getting a fitness tracker or glucose monitor to make tracking even easier. Whatever method you choose, make sure to be consistent and update your progress regularly. By doing so, you will set yourself up for success on your prediabetes diet journey.

Revamping your diet to follow a prediabetes nutrition plan is a great way to get on track for better health and keep your blood sugar levels in check. By following these steps, you can prepare yourself for taking on the challenge of making healthier lifestyle choices and ensuring that this prediabetes diet becomes part of a sustainable routine down the line. The key to success lies in understanding beneficial foods, creating meal plans and grocery lists, tracking progress, and making adjustments as necessary. With the right mindset, you'll be able to reap the rewards of a successful dietary change with ease!

HOW DIET AFFECTS PREDIABETES

Now that you know the basics of creating a prediabetes diet, it's time to look at how this type of diet can help those living with prediabetes. A healthy eating plan is essential for managing blood sugar levels and reducing your risk of developing diabetes or other health complications. With the right combination of foods, exercise, and lifestyle changes, you can begin to see real improvements in your overall health.

The focus of this guide is on diet. Why is that the case? How does diet affect prediabetes in the first place?

Losing weight and controlling your blood pressure and cholesterol levels are also linked to developing prediabetes. A lot of what you eat affects whether you develop prediabetes or not. Carbohydrates especially are strongly associated with a high blood sugar level.

So, how does it work? Taking a bite of a donut will surely not make you suddenly develop prediabetes. It can, only if your levels are already alarmingly high. The development of prediabetes or diabetes relies upon a diet that is consistently high in refined and processed sugars. It is not something that happens overnight. This is why when you get a diagnosis of prediabetes, it is important to take action right away.

When choosing foods, you have to consider the following:

Portion control

A piece of candy will not hurt you if you are not yet in the prediabetes or diabetes stage. So, how much of the prevention depends on portion control? Make sure that you stop eating when you are full. There is a tendency for some people to finish meals even when they are already full. The large portions of American meals are certainly not helping. A cup of a food item from years ago is more accurate.

Now, what they consider to be one cup or one serving is probably equivalent to two cups, instead. You may be tricked into taking in more than you planned to. Perhaps you can share with a family member or with a friend when you go out. At home, you can be stricter with your portions, with the use of measuring cups and even a food scale.

Daily requirement

Not everyone is expected to eat the same amount every day. A typical adult may be prescribed a 2200-calorie daily diet. If you are overweight, you may be advised to take fewer calories daily. However, being given a 2200-calorie total limit is not an excuse to binge on 2200 calories worth of carbohydrates.

Note that for those who are taking 2000 calories daily, a carbohydrate diet that ranges from 900 to 1300 calories is ideal. Unfortunately, this is not what is happening in reality. Carbohydrate sources are usually less expensive and more easily prepared and they tend to take over your daily intake. While it may be hard, try to stick to the recommended carbs.

Fiber in bulk

Fiber is not only good for your digestive system, but it also makes you feel full faster. This way, you will stop eating sooner than you would normally do. Just ask someone who has been eating a diet of brown rice instead of white rice. Brown rice, being unrefined and rich in fiber, can make you feel full fast. Processed and refined carbohydrates, on the other hand, are linked to many diseases. They are also stripped of their fiber and nutrients.

Staying sober

It is not just eating that can serve you up with your carbohydrates. Alcoholic beverages also contain quite a bit of carbohydrates. So, you will notice that if you drink a lot of beer, you may add a lot of weight. A lot of the beer weight also goes around your belly. Remember this is the most dangerous type of excess fat. Alcoholic beverages and sodas both contain a lot of sugars and must be imbibed in moderation if not completely taken out of the equation.

Hydration

While alcoholic drinks dehydrate, water hydrates. You know this since you were little. This is something that should be automatic: drinking a lot of water daily. Drinking plenty of water—aka hydrating—also helps lower blood sugar levels. The amount of water that you drink will depend on your weight, activity, and the number of sugary drinks that you drink daily. Just four of those eight-ounce servings of water can already improve your sugar level. However, do not wait for really high blood sugar levels (hyperglycemia) before you do something about it.

Benefits

Having a healthy diet is one of the best ways to prevent prediabetes and diabetes. Eating better will help you keep your blood sugar levels in check, avoid weight gain, and reduce your risk for chronic diseases. But it takes more than just cutting out refined and processed sugars.

You can reduce your risk of developing diabetes and other complications by following a prediabetes diet. Here are some of the benefits:

1. Lower Blood Sugar Levels: A prediabetes diet helps to regulate your blood sugar and keep it in check. Eating more fiber, whole grains, and non-starchy vegetables while avoiding processed

carbohydrates, sugary foods, and saturated fats helps to keep your blood sugar levels stable.

2. Improved Heart Health: Following a prediabetes diet lowers your risk for heart disease by reducing excessive cholesterol, triglycerides, and homocysteine levels in your blood. You can also benefit from exercising regularly on this diet as physical activity helps keep your heart healthy.

3. Weight Loss: A prediabetes diet can help you lose weight by decreasing the number of calories and unhealthy fats you consume, boosting your metabolism, and making better food choices that provide essential nutrients to your body. This in turn can help lower the risk of prediabetes from becoming diabetes or other health complications related to obesity.

4. Increased Energy Levels: Following a prediabetes diet improves overall energy levels due to healthier eating habits that provide essential vitamins and minerals to power our body's cells and organs efficiently. Eating a balanced meal of lean proteins, complex carbohydrates, fresh fruits, and vegetables will keep you energized throughout the day without feeling sluggish afterward.

5. Reduced Risk of Diabetes: The main goal of a prediabetes diet is to reduce blood sugar levels and the risk of developing Type 2 diabetes. Following this diet can help you maintain healthy blood glucose levels for those with pre-diabetes, which has been linked to reducing the risk of developing Type 2 diabetes in later life.

6. Improved Digestion: Eating foods that are high in fiber will help keep your digestive system functioning properly and can even reduce your risk for certain types of cancer. Fiber helps regulate bowel movements and keeps things moving along smoothly, so it's an important part of any diet plan—especially for those with prediabetes or diabetes.

7. Lower Blood Pressure: Prediabetes diets have been linked to lowering blood pressure when coupled with exercise and other lifestyle changes such as quitting smoking or reducing alcohol

consumption. Healthy eating habits help promote a healthy weight that reduces stress on the heart and vessels, thus improving overall cardiac health while helping regulate blood pressure levels.

8. Improved Cholesterol Levels: Eating a prediabetes diet can help reduce the number of unhealthy fats and cholesterol in your diet, which in turn can help lower your risk for heart-related issues. Foods such as nuts, avocados, and olive oil are great sources of healthy fats that can help reduce bad cholesterol levels in the body while providing essential nutrients like omega-3 fatty acids.

9. Enhanced Mental Health: Following a prediabetes diet can also help to improve mental health by reducing stress levels and inflammation associated with poor nutrition. Eating foods that contain essential vitamins, minerals, and antioxidants helps to boost serotonin production—a neurotransmitter responsible for regulating mood and emotions. Eating a balanced diet can positively impact overall mental health and help you feel more energized each day!

Making wise food choices can be hard at first but with the right knowledge and practice, it can become second nature. Knowing how much to eat, what types of foods to choose from, and how often you should drink water are only some of the considerations when choosing what kind of foods to put in your body. By taking these factors into account and maintaining a balanced diet, you can reap many health benefits such as improved energy levels, reduced risk for diseases such as diabetes or heart disease, and increased mental clarity & focus among others.

Cons
While a prediabetes diet can be beneficial to overall health, it is important to note that there are some downsides as well. Here are some of the cons of following a prediabetes diet that you might want to consider:

1. It can be restrictive: Restricting your food choices and

monitoring portion sizes can be a challenge when following a prediabetes diet. You'll need to become much more mindful of what you eat, which can be time-consuming and frustrating. In addition, you may need to cut back on some of your favorite foods, such as sweets and carbohydrate-rich dishes, to maintain healthy blood glucose levels. This can be a difficult adjustment to make, especially when you're used to indulging in these types of snacks and meals.

2. It can be difficult to stick to long-term: Making healthy food choices and sticking to a prediabetes diet can be difficult for some individuals. It requires dedication and commitment, which may become difficult to maintain over time. Also, unhealthy habits such as skipping meals or overeating can quickly undo any progress that has been made. If you find yourself having difficulty adhering to the diet long-term, it may be beneficial to speak with a dietician or nutritionist who can assist you in creating an eating plan that works for you.

3. It can be expensive: Eating healthier and following a prediabetes diet can often involve buying more expensive food items such as fresh fruits and vegetables, lean proteins, and whole grain products. While these foods can provide important nutrients, they may not always be cost-effective. To help reduce costs, consider buying in bulk or meal prepping to save time and money in the long run.

4. It's time-consuming: Monitoring your blood glucose levels regularly is an important part of managing prediabetes. While it can be beneficial to track progress and adjust your diet if necessary, this process can take up a lot of time. You'll need to schedule regular appointments with your healthcare provider and use a blood glucose meter to measure levels at home. You may need to take additional supplements or medications when following a prediabetes diet, which can be difficult to keep track of.

5. May be difficult to adjust to a healthy lifestyle: If you find it difficult to adjust your lifestyle to incorporate healthier habits,

following a prediabetes diet can pose a con for you. The changes that come with a prediabetes diet can be hard to stick to, as it requires you to eliminate unhealthy foods and replace them with healthier alternatives. This may be particularly challenging if you are used to eating high-carbohydrate or sugary foods that you enjoy. Furthermore, following a prediabetes diet may take more effort and require more planning than your previous eating habits, which can be a burden for those with busy schedules or limited cooking skills.

6. Risk of developing deficiencies in essential vitamins, minerals, and other nutrients: If you are following a prediabetes diet, you may want to be cautious about the potential risks of nutrient deficiencies. When you cut out certain foods or food groups, you may inadvertently miss out on crucial vitamins, minerals, and other nutrients your body needs. For example, if you limit your carbohydrate intake, you may not be getting enough fiber, which is important for digestive health. Additionally, low-carb diets may lead to a decreased intake of some B vitamins, which are essential for energy production and overall metabolic health. To mitigate the risk of nutrient deficiencies, it is important to talk to a healthcare professional, monitor your nutrient intake, and choose a balanced and varied diet that provides all the essential nutrients your body needs.

Overall, the cons of following a prediabetes diet should be carefully weighed against the potential benefits—but with some dedication and care, this lifestyle change can help manage your condition and associated symptoms.

BEST FOODS FOR PREDIABETES

At this point, you know what you should be avoiding. You also know what you should be ingesting quite a bit of (water, fiber). How about if the list gets more specific? This chapter is dedicated to specific foods that you should add to your grocery list next time if you haven't bought them yet.

Hyperglycemia is mostly affected by carbohydrates. So, your first step is to look for foods that do not have or have very little of this food group.

Take a look at some zero-carb foods:
Oils, butter, meat, and eggs have zero carbs

If you are still familiar with your food groups, you will recognize these as mostly protein-rich foods. They will help you build up your body and protect your immune system without packing in the carbs. However, you should also remind yourself that fats can also affect prediabetes. If you take in too much red meat and oils, for example, you are at risk of developing high cholesterol and hypertension. These conditions are also linked to prediabetes. These zero-carb foods, in moderation, are otherwise perfect for your prediabetes diet. They can also be quite savory: just a note for those who are worrying about a prediabetes diet (or any diet for that matter!) can be boring.

How about some low-carb foods?
Tofu, nuts, seeds, non-starchy veggies, yogurt, avocados, and cheese are just some examples of low-carb foods.

Now, you are getting somewhere. These are quite an interesting bunch and the list has something for everyone. These are mostly low-fat and low-carb foods at the same time. Avocados provide good cholesterol, which the body needs because it helps get rid of bad cholesterol.

This list also includes foods that are very easy to prepare and serve. Part of the concern about diets lies in the preparation. Sometimes, some of the foods can be fussy to prepare and expensive to buy.

Then, should you also include medium carb content?
Beans, peas, lentils, and berries all fall under this category.

Medium carb content can change things from time to time. You may be surprised that some vegetables fall under this category. Fruits, of course, have their share of sugars. Berries are comparatively safer than other fruits, such as mangoes.

You may add the foods from this list from time to time. Beans, peas, and lentils may make you full quickly enough before you overload your carbohydrate limit.

Other low-carb foods that you may consider:
- Spinach
- Tomatoes
- Asparagus
- Zucchini
- Lettuce
- Carrots
- Celery

There is more, but you are getting the idea.

Foods that are high in carbohydrates are, unfortunately, not easy to give up. They tend to be tasty and attractive. The reason a lot of children are developing obesity and diabetes at a very young age is that plenty of fast food restaurants offer delicious but high-carb, high-fat foods, such as French fries, fried chicken rolled in a lot of flour, cakes, and the like.

As a whole, when deciding if a particular food has high carbohydrate content, what you are interested in is the Glycemic Index (GI). GI is used to provide you with a quick look at whether a food item is good for you if you already have prediabetes.

Here are a few examples of foods and their corresponding GIs.
• Fruit Roll-Ups (99)
• Cornflakes (93)
• White Spaghetti (58)
• Wholemeal spaghetti (42)
• Watermelon (72)
• Apple (39)

These are very few, but they can already give you an idea that some things are not what they seem. Everybody knows that Fruit Roll-Ups have plenty of sugar, but the use of the word "fruit" can be deceiving. People may think it is healthy. If you have eaten one, you will notice that it can be too sweet but does not fill you. You end up finishing several, racking more of the GIs.

Cornflakes are also advertised as part of a healthy breakfast, but they may not be that healthy for someone with prediabetes.

The GI comparison between the two types of spaghetti drives home the fact that refined carbohydrates are unhealthy, compared to their rougher, fiber-rich counterparts.

Even fresh fruits can be a problem. You have been taught to eat your fruits and veggies. Do be careful about what kind you are eating.

PREDIABETES DIETS TO CONSIDER

You may have picked this guide because you have been newly diagnosed with prediabetes or you are just starting to go on the road to healthy eating. So, you will be presented with some of the simplest prediabetes diets out there. There is no need to pay a nutritionist to provide you with guidance. You just need a notebook (electronic or paper-based) to record what you have been eating, a pen, and the Internet. The Internet will provide you with the numbers that you will need when calculating calories or GIs.

Traditional Meal Planning versus Eating Out

If you plan to cook at home, the best thing to do first is to go shopping. Buy the foods that you like from the zero-carb, low-carb, and medium-carb categories. Find out their GIs and calorie content. You can devise your daily diet table. If you do not have a lot of time to think about meals for every single day of the year, you can repeat the same setup every Monday. You can have Nuts and Fish Monday, for example. You can change a detail at a time to keep things interesting.

What you will need:
- Internet
- Food scale

- Calculator
- Record keeper (laptop or an actual notebook)

An example of a balanced prediabetes menu (for one day) goes like this:

Breakfast
- 1/2 cup oatmeal, in skim milk
- A low-fat yogurt
- An ounce of nuts

Lunch:
- Tuna melt

Dinner:
- Baked salmon

As for eating out, yes you can do that. You do have to keep away from fast food restaurants. Find a restaurant known for serving low-calorie items. Emphasize that you have a health issue that must be taken seriously.

Plate Method

If you want a quicker prediabetes diet, then you can pick the plate method. You only need to remember that you will need:
- A quarter of fish, meat, or another source of protein
- Quarter carbs, such as potatoes, rice, pasta, or bread (They are not completely banned!)
- Two servings of half-cup veggies
- A low or medium-carb fruit
- Water or any other low-calorie drink

You can keep changing the contents of your plate as you see fit.

From what you have just read, there is no need to live a boring life just because you have decided to go on a healthier path.

BONUS RECIPES

Stir-Fried Chicken and Veggies

Ingredients:
- 2 green onions, cut into quarter-inch thick
- 2 carrots, sliced thinly into rounds
- 1 lb. chicken breast, boneless, skinless, and cut into strips
- 1 zucchini, medium-sized, cut into half moon, about a quarter of an inch thick
- 2 cups broccoli florets
- 4 garlic cloves, minced
- 1 jalapeño pepper, seeds removed and minced
- 1/4 cup fresh cilantro, chopped
- 1/4 cup fresh basil, sliced
- 1 tbsp. fresh ginger, minced
- 2 tbsp. reduced-sodium soy sauce, divided
- 1 lime, juice only, divided
- 2 tsp. sesame oil, divided
- 1 tbsp. expeller pressed canola oil
- optional: brown rice

Instructions:
1. In a large bowl or plastic bag with a zip-top, put the ginger, a teaspoon of sesame oil, half of the lime juice, and a tablespoon of soy sauce. Combine everything by mixing or shaking well.
2. Add the chicken to the marinade and coat it well.
3. Seal the bag or cover the bowl and keep it in the fridge for at least an hour and up to 24 hours.
4. Place a large nonstick skillet or wok over medium-high heat. Heat up the oil.
5. Pour the marinated chicken with its sauce to stir-fry for a minute.
6. Follow it up with the following: broccoli, carrots, garlic, green onions, jalapeno pepper, and zucchini. Stir-fry until the vegetables are crisp and tender and the chicken is cooked through for about 7 minutes.
7. Add the remaining ingredients, lime juice, sesame oil, and soy

sauce. Mix well.
8. Mix in the basil and cilantro before serving.
9. If desired, serve with brown rice.

Pickled Asparagus

Ingredients:
- 1 lb. fresh asparagus, trim the ends and cut into preferred lengths and wash well
- 1/4 cup cider vinegar
- 1/4 cup pearl onions
- 1 sprig of fresh dill, or 2 tsp. if dried
- 1/4 cup white wine vinegar
- 8 whole black peppercorns
- 3 cloves garlic
- 1/4 tsp. red pepper flakes
- 1 cup water
- 6 whole coriander seeds

Instructions:
1. In air-tight containers, combine all the ingredients.
2. Refrigerate for up to 4 weeks.

Tomato Crostini

Ingredients:
- 4 plum tomatoes, chopped
- 1/4 lb. toasted Italian peasant bread, sliced into 4
- 1 clove garlic, minced
- 1/4 cup fresh basil, minced
- freshly ground pepper
- 2 tsp. olive oil

Instructions:
1. In a bowl, combine basil, garlic, oil, pepper, and tomatoes.
2. Cover it and leave for half an hour.
3. Serve by spreading the mixture on the toast.

Baked Chicken and Wild Rice with Onions and Tarragon

Ingredients:
- 1 lb. boneless, skinless chicken breast halves, cut into 1-inch slices
- 2 cups unsalted chicken broth, divided
- 1 1/2 cups celery, chopped
- 1 1/2 cups pearl onions, whole
- 1 1/2 cups dry white wine
- 3/4 cup uncooked long-grain white rice
- 3/4 cup uncooked wild rice
- 1 tsp. fresh tarragon

Instructions:
1. Preheat the oven to 300°F.
2. Place a non-stick frying pan over medium heat and cook the chicken with onion, tarragon, celery, and a cup of broth for about 10 minutes, or until everything is tender. Set aside.
3. Grab a baking dish to stir the rice, wine, and remaining broth. Leave it to soak for half an hour.
4. Put the chicken and veggies into the baking dish, cover, and bake for an hour.
5. Check the chicken from time to time, and pour broth to keep the rice from drying out.
6. Once done, serve immediately.

Grilled Salmon

Ingredients:
- 2 4-oz. salmon filets
- 1/2 tsp. salt
- 1/2 tsp. black pepper
- vegetable cooking spray

Instructions:
1. Prep a cast-iron skillet or a grill over medium heat and spray cooking spray.
2. Use the cooking spray also on the salmon filets, on both sides. Then season one side with pepper and salt.
3. Put the seasoned side of the fillet on the grill to cook for 3 minutes. Do the same on the other side.
4. Once done, serve and enjoy.

<u>**Spanish Omelet**</u>

Ingredients:
- 3 whole eggs, beaten
- 5 egg whites, beaten
- 3 oz. part-skim mozzarella cheese, shredded
- 5 small potatoes, peeled and sliced
- 1/2 medium onion, minced
- 1 small zucchini, sliced
- 1 tbsp. low-fat parmesan cheese
- 5 medium mushrooms, sliced
- 1-1/2 cups green or red peppers, thinly sliced
- Pepper, garlic, salt with herbs, to taste
- vegetable cooking spray

Instructions:
1. Preheat the oven to 375°F.
2. Boil a pot of water to cook the potatoes until tender. Set aside once done.
3. Spray veggie spray on a nonstick pan placed over medium heat.
4. Sauté onion until brown.
5. Follow it up with the veggies until everything is well cooked.
6. In a bowl, beat the eggs and egg whites slightly. Add the seasoning and the cheese.
7. Pour the egg-cheese mixture into the pan and stir-fry everything.
8. In a baking dish or skillet, prep with vegetable spray. Put the stir-fried veggies, egg mixture, and drained potatoes in the dish.
9. Sprinkle with cheese and bake for 20-30 minutes, or until the top is brown and firm.
10. Once done, cool for 10 minutes before serving.

<u>**Two Cheese Pizza**</u>

Ingredients:
- 1 10-oz. can refrigerated pizza crust
- 1 large red pepper, cut into strips
- 4 oz. part-skim mozzarella cheese, shredded
- 2 cups mushrooms, chopped
- 1/2 cup low-fat ricotta cheese
- 2 tbsp. whole wheat flour
- 2 tbsp. olive oil
- 1/2 tsp. dried basil
- 2 garlic cloves, minced
- 1 small onion, minced
- vegetable cooking spray
- optional: 1/4 tsp. salt

Instructions:
1. Preheat the oven to 425°F.
2. Prep the surface by dusting it with flour.
3. Roll the dough on the dusted surface with a rolling pin. Keep rolling until you get your desired crust thickness.
4. Prep a cookie sheet by spraying cooking spray before transferring the pizza crust to the sheet. Then, apply olive oil to the crust with a brush.
5. In a bowl, mix the two types of cheeses. Distribute this mixture on the crust evenly.
6. Top it with the mushroom, garlic, onion, basil, and red pepper. Season with salt.
7. Pop in the oven and bake until the crust is golden.

Fruity Yogurt

Ingredients:
- 8 oz. fat-free, sugar-free orange yogurt
- 3 oz. or 1/2 cup honeydew melon, cubed
- 3 oz. or 1/2 cup watermelon, cubed and seeds removed
- 3 oz. or 1/2 cup cantaloupe melon, cubed
- 1/2 cup unsweetened orange juice
- 1 mango, cubed, peeled, and seeded
- 1 papaya, cubed, peeled, and seeded
- 2 pcs. oranges, sliced and seeded
- 5 strawberries, cut into halves

Instructions:
1. Mix the fruits and yogurt in a bowl.
2. Pour orange juice over the fruit mixture.
3. Mix well and serve.

Low-Fat Buttermilk Panna Cotta with Peaches

Ingredients:
- 2 cups buttermilk
- 400g sliced peaches
- 2 tsp. powdered gelatin
- 1 vanilla bean
- 2 tbsp. caster sugar

Instructions:
1. Put buttermilk, vanilla bean, and sugar in a saucepan and stir occasionally over medium-low heat until well heated through but without reaching simmering or boiling level. This should take around six to eight minutes.
2. Remove the saucepan from the heat.
3. Strain heated ingredients into a bowl
4. Add in gelatin powder and whisk until fully dissolved
5. Let the mixture cool for 10 minutes
6. Meanwhile, while waiting for the mixture to cool down, prepare the panna cotta molds by lightly greasing them.
7. Pour the cooled mixture into the mold and cover it with plastic wrap
8. Refrigerate the covered mold for four hours or until set.
9. Once set, turn out panna cotta onto a serving plate and garnish with sliced peaches

<u>**Sugar-free Chocolate Muffins**</u>

Ingredients:
Muffin:
- 50g sugar-free milk chocolate, chopped
- 1.5 cups plain flour
- 2 eggs
- 1 cup buttermilk
- ½ cup stevia for baking
- ¼ cup cacao powder
- 3 teaspoons baking powder
- 100ml macadamia oil
- 1 teaspoon pure vanilla extract

Icing:
- 1 large peeled and seeded ripe avocado
- 2 tablespoons of sifted cocoa powder
- Liquid stevia, to taste

Instructions:
1. Preheat oven to 180c
2. Line muffin tin with very lightly greased paper cases
3. Sift flour, cacao, and baking powder in a large bowl
4. Add in stevia and mix well
5. In a separate bowl, whisk together the buttermilk, eggs, vanilla extract, and macadamia oil until well blended.
6. Pour the wet ingredients mixture into the bowl of dry ingredients mixture and combine well
7. Stir in chopped chocolate
8. Pour the mixture into prepared muffin cups and bake for 20 minutes or until golden.
9. Once baked, take it out from the oven and allow the muffins to cool down.
10. While waiting for the muffins to cool down, prepare the icing.
11. Put all icing ingredients in a food processor and process until completely smooth.
12. Spread icing evenly on the tops of the cooled muffins.

CONCLUSION

Thank you for taking the time to learn about prediabetes, diabetes, and prediabetes diet. By now, we hope that you have a better understanding of these conditions and how you can take preventive measures to reduce the risk of developing type 2 diabetes. We also hope that this guide has given you an introduction to some important tips on incorporating healthy dietary habits into your lifestyle.

Living with prediabetes doesn't have to be intimidating or overwhelming. Making small changes in your day-to-day life, such as watching portion sizes and engaging in regular physical activity, can help you reduce insulin resistance and maintain an active lifestyle. With the right approach, prediabetes can turn into a manageable condition rather than something to fear.

Most importantly, please remember that there is no one-size-fits-all approach when it comes to managing prediabetes or diabetes. Everyone's body is unique and what works for one person may not work for another. It's important to consult with your doctor about any medical concerns so they can provide personalized advice for your particular situation.

We thank you again for taking the time to read through this guide and wish you success in your journey toward health and well-being.

REFERENCES AND HELPFUL LINKS

7 diet tips for people with prediabetes. (2014, August 21). Healthline. https://www.healthline.com/health/diabetes/prediabetes-diet.

About diabetes. (2014, August 6). Congressional Diabetes Caucus. https://diabetescaucus-degette.house.gov/facts-and-figures.

CDC. (2021, December 21). Prediabetes—Your chance to prevent type 2 diabetes. Centers for Disease Control and Prevention. http://bit.ly/2hMpYrt.

CNBC.com, L. K., special to. (2017, August 31). One third of Americans are headed for diabetes, and they don't even know it. CNBC. https://www.cnbc.com/2017/08/31/type-2-diabetes-may-hit-84-million-americans-and-they-dont-know-it.html.

Prediabetes diet. (2022, October 31). https://www.hopkinsmedicine.org/health/wellness-and-prevention/prediabetes-diet.

Prediabetes—Symptoms and causes. (n.d.). Mayo Clinic. Retrieved April 15, 2023, from https://www.mayoclinic.org/diseases-conditions/prediabetes/symptoms-causes/syc-20355278.

www.ingramcontent.com/pod-product-compliance
Lightning Source LLC
Chambersburg PA
CBHW051126250726
48655CB00007B/2903